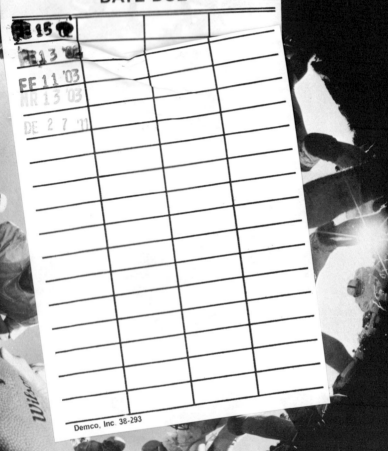

DATE DUE

YOGA CONDITIONING AND FOOTBALL

by

JERRY COLLETTO

Chairman, P.E. Department and Head J.V. Coach

Novato High School

Novato, California

with
Jack L. Sloan, Ed.D.

Photos
by
Lun Yun Ng

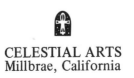

CELESTIAL ARTS
Millbrae, California

First Printing, August 1975
Made in the United States of America

Library of Congress Cataloging in Publication Data

Colletto, Jerry, 1940-
    Yoga conditioning & football.

    1. Football--Training. 2. Yoga, Hatha. I. Sloan,
Jack L., joint author. II. Title.
GV951.C64   613.7   75-9439
ISBN 0-89087-018-7

To my wife Kathy and my sons Steven and Christopher

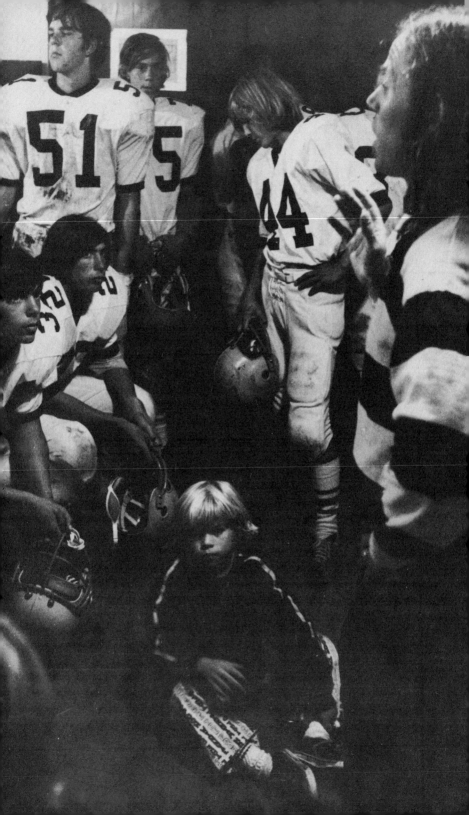

Table of Contents

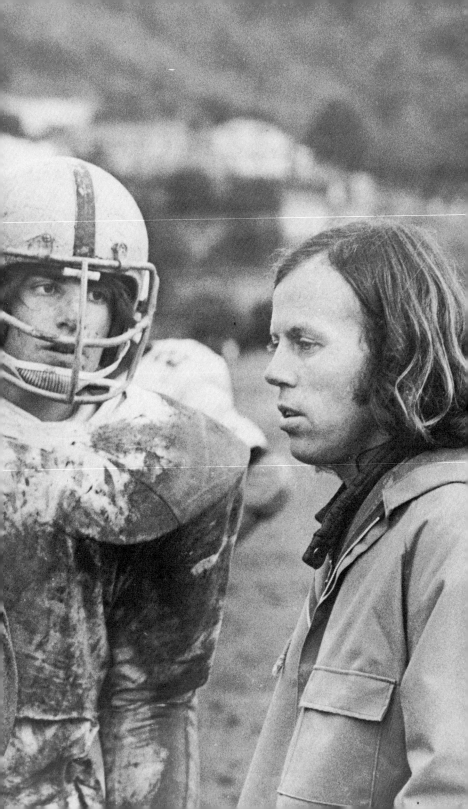

Preface

This book represents four years of experimenting, studying, practicing and putting together a new concept of conditioning. The method we use has proved to be very beneficial to our program, and also to improving ourselves.

In the four years of using the Yoga techniques we have not had a player miss a game due to a muscle pull injury. As a person concerned about injuries in athletics, I would like to share my ideas with you.

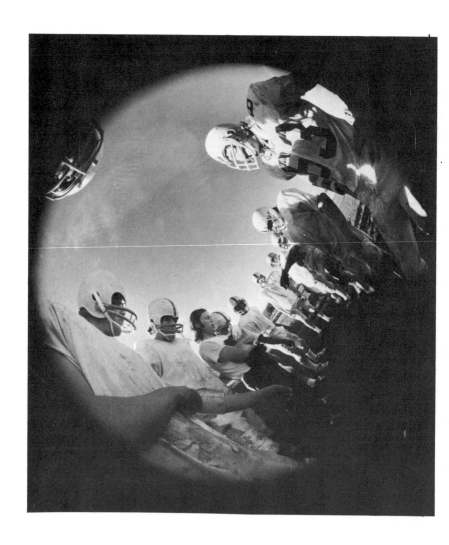

1

An Introduction to Yoga Conditioning

Injuries have always been a problem in strenuous sports. This has been particularly true of football. When I was in high school the parents of several of my friends would not let their sons participate because of fear of injury. Many older people who have participated in athletics still complain of injuries suffered on playing fields years before. Even professional athletes are concerned. One of the items on the 1974 agenda of the National Football League was the injury problem.

This book was written with the intention of helping coaches and players prevent injuries through better conditioning. It is intended to have value for all sports, not just football. However, I am a football coach and I use the techniques in this book with my players. I find that it is easier for me to express my feelings through football.

I'm not trying to suggest that hatha yoga is a cure-all for your conditioning problems. Hatha yoga may not even be a valuable technique for you personally to use in any way. It predates modern football by almost 5,000 years and we have reason to believe that those who designed the exercises we discuss here did not have any athletes and athletics in mind. Yet we find the conditioning provided by hatha yoga to be beneficial to our team. I think that if you try the conditioning program I describe here, or even only a small part of it, you will find the results interesting. If it will be good to you, it will come to you.

Even though yoga as a science of the physical, mental, and spiritual body is thousands of years old, it has really only become popular in this country over the past decade. Yoga as a science is designed to serve its own ends, and its merits some inquiry and study for its own sake. We advocate taking only a small part of the yoga tradition and adopting it to suit modern American sports.

Hatha yoga is that branch of yoga which deals with our physical bodies. The positions we describe are traditionally called asanas. We often refer to them here as exercises.

The style of hatha yoga exercises provides a contrast to exercises in the usual athletic conditioning program. It is important to do these exercises slowly and gracefully. We never rush or throw ourselves aggressively into a yoga posture. Instead, we move thoughtfully, each person at his or her own pace. There is no sense of competition in our yoga conditioning workouts. We each accept the differences among us in our ability to stretch or bend in new ways. As we progress through weeks and months of practice, we are delighted and even amazed at the way our bodies change. One way to characterize the spirit would be to say we become more aware of ourselves as we progress.

The pace of a hatha yoga conditioning session is important. After each exercise it is a good practice to relax on your back or stomach, or at least to breathe deeply a few times. Rest periods let the part of the body which was just used recover from its activity. Sometimes the person exercising can almost feel the benefit of the exercise settling into the body during the rest times.

In a setting, such as a physical education class or at home, more time can be taken to relax between asanas, but in a conditioning session which is only one part of a sports practice period, time is often at a premium. When time is an important factor, relax as often as possible. The *right* pace and *right* combination of exercise will come with experience and is a matter of personal taste. To help you get started, we have suggested a daily workout schedule in the last chapter of this book.

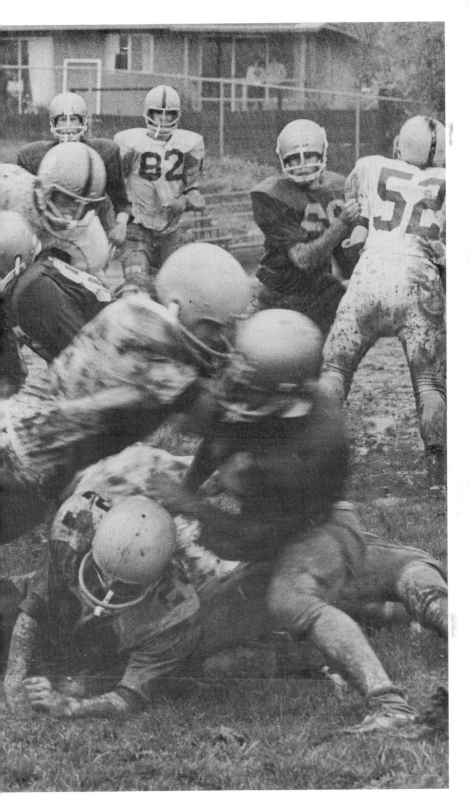

I have been a student of hatha yoga for five years. While I don't feel I can recommend myself as an expert on yoga, I do believe that the techniques described in this book may help you to use your body at its fullest potential. My experience indicates that yoga promotes flexibility of the spine and muscles, quickness, agility, balance, mental concentration, coordination and strength. Cardiovascular endurance is improved by the breathing techniques and internal organs improve in their functioning as well. If you wish to learn more about the more esoteric benefits of yoga, there are many excellent books available. Instruction by a qualified yoga teacher is the best way to any but superficial knowledge.

In teaching any team sport, a coach finds that there is a real limit on how many drills, patterns, and formations a player can profitably learn. If you study your sport carefully, you'll realize that knowing the techniques that are in style in any given season is only part of the mental skills necessary to win. The other part is concentration. In my view, the key to successful teaching or coaching is in helping the player to concentrate, to remember what he has learned, to eliminate mistakes. An athlete can remember occasions when a key assignment was missed or a silly mistake was made. If we are able to intensify our concentration, many of these mistakes can be eliminated.

Yoga seems to me to provide a way to increase concentration. Breathing offers the key. During each of the exercises we discuss here we advocate a certain type of breathing. We call it abdominal breathing, explained in some detail in the next chapter. We urge people who are doing yoga exercises to concentrate on the feeling and sound of their breathing and on the particular part of the body on which the exercise works. By breathing in deeply and relaxing when exhaling, often a muscle will stretch or flex a little bit more. Once a person observes this in his or her own body, it is easier to keep the attention focused on the exercise.

Focusing attention on a specific object, even a part of your own body, in a calm and still environment, sets a kind of tone for a practice session or a game day. Moving thoughtfully to a posture which then is held while concentration is focused through controlled, deep breathing is far different than the traditional football warm-up. Most western calisthenics are performed as short, jerky movements accompanied by shallow mouth breathing. The resulting frenetic atmosphere detracts from concentration and provides little in the way of loosening up of muscles and minds.

Dave Meggesey in his book *Out of Their League* reports an experience I'm sure many athletes share. He says that often he would get so worked up before a game that he felt like a wild animal. He claims that he frequently had to compensate with brutal aggressiveness for forgotten plays and poorly executed assignments.

This certainly provides a contrast to the kind of player I hope to develop. Instead of spending energy "getting up" for the game, we try to focus our attention on our bodies. Instead of panting through our mouths, we breathe deeply through our noses. Instead of jumping and plunging, we settle into our asanas stretching and concentrating. Instead of frantic emotional outbursts, we are prepared to think clearly and calmly before we act.

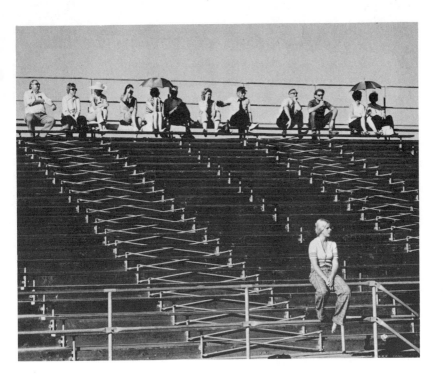

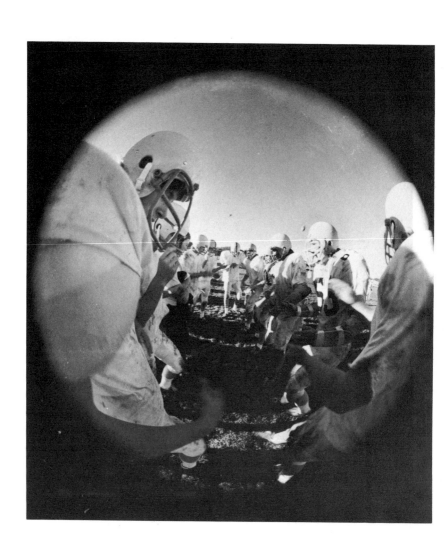

2

Yoga Breathing, Yoga
on the Field and Yoga Attitude

This chapter is devoted to some basic aspects of our application of yoga to football at the school where I coach. One of those aspects is the yoga perspective on breathing and implications it has for a strenuous sport like football. Another aspect centers on the way we apply parts of the yoga way to our behavior on the field, in practice and in games. The third aspect deals with our attempts to employ a yoga like attitude in the way we relate to each other as people as well as the way we play the sport.

Breathing. In yoga we learn a controlled way of breathing which has many functions. We have already briefly discussed the role of breathing in training for better concentration. A slow and controlled way of breathing affects changes in other systems in the body beyond the respiratory system. Slow, deep breaths tend to slow the heart and place less strain on the whole cardiovascular system. Slow, deep breathing also adds extra oxygen to the metabolism process. This, in turn, promotes the consumption of fatty deposits and aids in the removal of diseased and used up cells. Extra oxygen to muscles, joints and organs makes for more energy. All of these effects can be achieved through yoga techniques. Yoga focuses on the breathing, probably because it is the more or less automatic process in the body which lends itself most readily to conscious control.

Yogis often say the mouth is for eating and talking, the nose is for breathing. Breaths taken through the mouth tend to be shallow and short. Typically, only the upper sections of the lungs are used. The nose filters and warms a breath. Those breaths take longer on the way in as well as on the way out. This provides extra exercise for the muscles for the breathing mechanism. A behavioral psychologist might note that nose breathing is more likely to happen when one is calm, or in repose. Thus, when we breathe through the nose we tend to be more calm. Mouth breathing is usually associated with excitement and even the loss of emotional control, as in sobbing. Thus, mouth breathing heightens our emotionality and correspondingly reduces the deliberateness of our actions.

The breathing technique which we generally use in our yoga conditioning sessions is called abdominal breathing. It stretches the lower lobes of the lungs and seems to calm and stabilize emotions. We start with a standing position, hands loosely at the sides. It is important to stand straight with the shoulders back and chin held high. The spine is straight, but not stiff. The air can then flow freely, deep into the lower parts of the lungs.

Try it yourself. Inhale by breathing slowly and steadily for several seconds through the nose. Let the stomach expand as far as possible, or until you cannot get any more air into the lungs. Then exhale slowly but steadily through the nose. Push the last bit of air out by collapsing the stomach in towards the spine.

You can check yourself to see if you are doing abdominal breathing correctly by putting one hand on your stomach and the other on your chest. As you breathe in and out, the hand on your stomach should move as we have indicated. The hand on your chest should remain still.

Two other breathing exercises might prove useful in conditioning sessions and in games.

Complete Breathing. This exercise provides a complete ventilation of the lungs. It tones the entire respiratory system. It gives the body renewed energy, and it helps you to catch your breath quickly after strenuous effort. We recommend this exercise for time-outs during games. In that context, it helps a player gather strength and relax mentally.

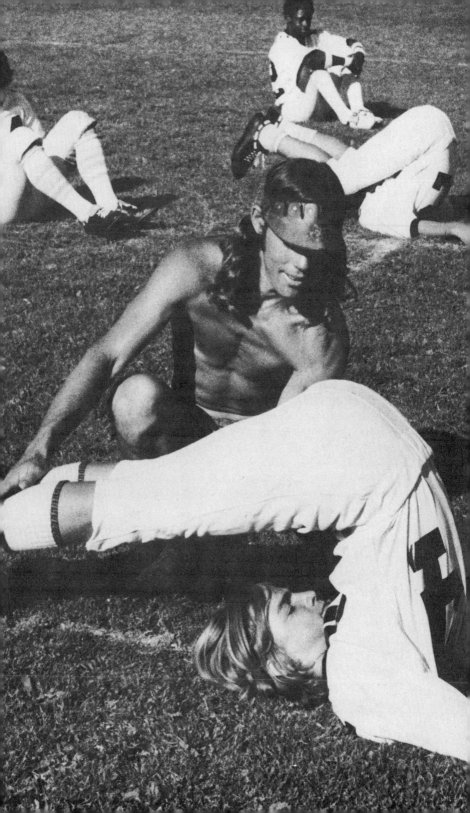

Instructions: Stand straight with shoulders back, head straight ahead and hands at your sides. Breathe slowly and steadily in through your nose only. First, let your stomach come out with the breath. Then, as the inhalation continues, suck your stomach in toward the spine and fill the chest cavity. Finally, still breathing in, raise your shoulders to fill the top portion of your lungs. Hold your breath for five or ten seconds and then exhale slowly and steadily through the nose.

Alternate Nostril Breathing. This exercise is particularly good for controlling the pregame jitters. Many athletes become tense while thinking about competing in an athletic event. Not everyone will agree, but we generally feel that this tension is a wasted energy that could be used to more advantage in the game. With this exercise it is possible to control nervous tension and conserve one's energy.

Instructions: Stand or sit with the shoulders back, back straight and the head facing forward. The left hand should rest at your side. Using the first finger of your right hand, close the left nostril of your nose. Now inhale slowly, steadily and deeply, filling the stomach as in abdominal breathing, through the right nostril. Then close the right nostril with your thumb and remove your finger from the side of the left nostril. Now exhale slowly, steadily and completely from the left nostril.

Now keep your thumb where it is and inhale through the left nostril. Then close the left nostril with your finger and exhale through the right nostril. That sequence is one round of breathing. Repeat the whole thing several times, or until you feel relaxed and alert.

Any of the breathing exercises can be done just as well while lying on your back. the posture we use is called the sponge position and it is discussed in detail in Chapter 8. the sponge is good to use before the game and during breaks between periods or halfs. We use this time to relax, gather energy from the air, and concentrate on our assignments in the game and the techniques we use.

There certainly is a lot more to learn about breathing in hatha yoga. These are just a few techniques which seem to have particular relevance to sports.

Yoga Conditioning at Football Practice. We spend at least 20 minutes a day on yoga conditioning, but yoga spirit is part of

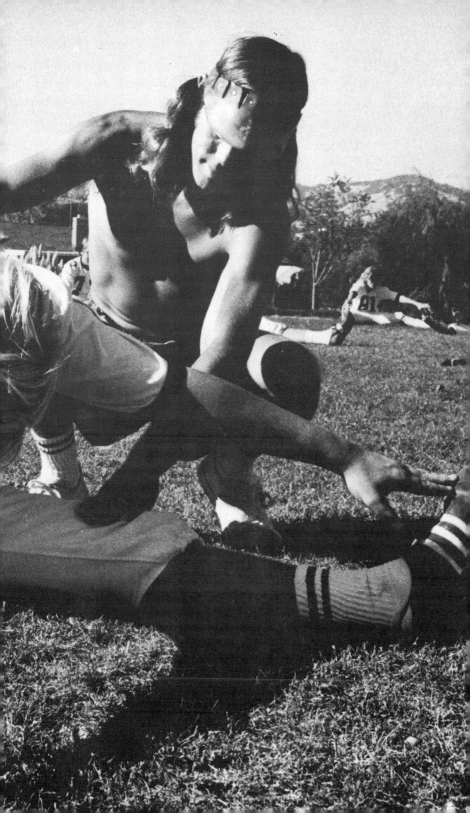

the whole practice session. We use yoga exercises to stretch and make our bodies flexible and strong at the beginning of practice. We then use yoga breathing throughout the practice and at the end we use yoga exercises to tone us down, eliminate soreness and get us ready to do the things we have to do besides football practice.

Common sense tells us that it isn't a good idea to eat just before football practice. This is especially true of yoga conditioning since yoga stretches and twists the internal organs including the digestive tract. We recommend no eating during the three hours before a yoga conditioning session. If a person must eat, we suggest something easily digestible like yogurt.

The less clothing one wears while doing yoga, the better. We recommend no shoes, if possible, and loose fitting clothing. At our yoga football conditioning sessions we wear shoes, but no shoulder pads or helmets.

There are probably over 2,000 variations of the basic yoga postures which can be learned and could be used in football conditioning. We use only 15 or 20 of these on any one day. We structure the conditioning sessions so that all parts of the body are stretched and worked, including the internal organs. In the last chapter we will discuss the way we work up a program of exercises for a specific practice session.

During practice we use yoga breathing to help concentrate on what is being taught and the proper execution of the lessons learned. That means that when a player is waiting in line to run a pass pattern, or block, or what have you, he is encouraged to concentrate on his breathing, breathe deeply into the abdomen using only the nose, and to consider what he is about to do with his body and mind. Total relaxation, total concentration and total oneness with the game is the goal.

When practice is over we usually take five or ten minutes to tone down. We use a couple of the more relaxed postures which, in my experience, counter soreness in the legs and back. We finish with a couple of minutes of just lying on the back and breathing deeply, concentrating on the breath passing in and out of the body.

In our huddle we stand up instead of bending over as most teams do. In the typical huddle the players, in a circle, lean over the quarterback who calls the next play. Most players breathe rapidly through the mouth while listening to the play. Mouth breathing is natural after heavy exertion and when one is bent over with the diaphragm collapsed.

Instead, we stand upright with our heads back. We try to encourage the players to breathe deeply, doing abdominal breathing. By standing in the huddle taking the deep breath and relaxing, our players can relax and concentrate on what the next play will be and what must be done to execute it in as nearly a perfect fashion as possible. They know that if they understand their role in the next play and execute perfectly, the play will work and eventually we will win.

Standing up straight also helps to maintain a confident, positive attitude. People who go around hump-shouldered and bent over, breathing shallowly are not really confident in themselves. People who are confident and positive about themselves go around with their heads up and shoulders back. By using a stand up straight posture in our huddles, we maximize our positive attitude through physical means.

I feel that in football a player must eventually learn to concentrate and focus his energy for the five or six seconds that the ball is in play. In the five or six seconds during which a play is run we want the maximum effort that our players can muster. We try to teach our players to relax in the huddle. Our thoughts about our techniques and assignments go deep. We relax and mentally run over what must be done. particularly, we try to teach our players to concentrate on exploding into action. We teach the contrast between relaxation as complete as the situation will allow and activity as intense as the player can make it.

Instead of standing around talking to their friends, our players in drill, and in the game, concentrate on their breathing and their techniques and assignments. Football is a game of mental concentration.

As practice goes on I try to emphasize keeping myself under control. When I am successful, it has an effect on the players. It gives them confidence and they come to trust me and feel together with me. I explain to them that we all make mistakes. Mistakes are things we don't worry about. We don't think about them but we try to eliminate mistakes.

We manage this by trying to forget the past and just being involved with the *now*. When a player worries about his mistakes,

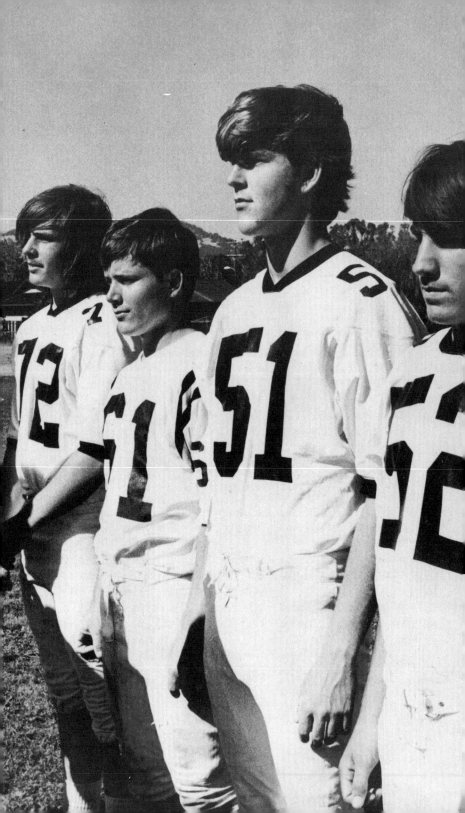

then they build up on him and keep him from doing the right thing on the next play.

My players know the coach doesn't get upset or angry about mistakes. What happens is immediately in the past, which frees us to concentrate on what is happening next.

Bob Aucone, my co-coach, and I have found that if we keep ourselves positive and open, then the players feel free to talk to us. Listening to the players has often provided valuable lessons for us. The more we know about what's happening on the field and off, the better we are able to lead the team.

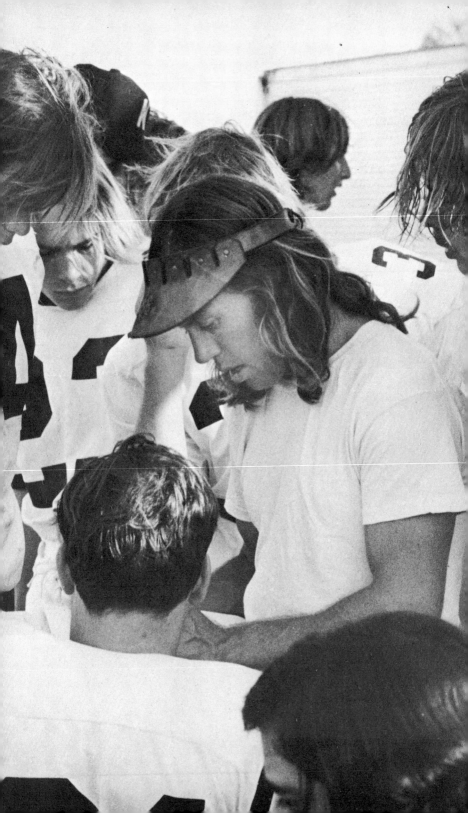

3

A General Warm-Up Exercise

In this chapter we will introduce the first of more than 30 exercises (asanas). Throughout the rest of the book we will discuss each exercise in a format that includes a brief discussion of the benefits and applications of the exercise, a detailed description of the way to do the exercise and a picture that shows how the exercise looks when you get into it.

We think the best way to use the parts of the book which describe the exercises is to actually do the exercises as you read. In that way you get the best possible idea about the way the exercise affects your body.

If you do decide to "work" your way through the next few chapters, then you should be aware of the same things Bob and I point out to the players at yoga work-outs on the practice field.

First, there is a lot of reference in the instructions to breathing. Every session that we do starts with a few abdominal breaths. Breathe only through your nose. Let your stomach loosen up and go out as you breathe in. Imagine the breath moving down inside you along your spinal column. Breathe slowly. Fill your body to its maximum. When you breathe out, let our stomach collapse. Be sure to breath all the air you possibly can back out. Try to keep your attention focused only on the sound and feel of your breathing.

As you will soon see, we start each description of an exercise with a discussion of the benefits that come from doing that exercise. In our discussion we often mention specific parts of the body. When we lead the players in yoga exercises on the field, we mention these parts of the body so the players can focus their attention on them as well as on their breathing. For instance, if the discussion says an exercise stretches the groin muscles, then concentrate on loosening and stretching the groin when you do the exercise. Here's a hint. Concentrate on stretching and loosening on outgoing breaths. Concentrate on moving and tightening on incoming breaths.

The salute to the sun, our first exercise, has eight separate postures within it. therefore, we have devoted the rest of the chapter to it. The other exercises we do are considerably less complex.

Exercise: Salute to the Sun

Benefits: This exercise promotes movement of the spine and stretches various ligaments and muscles in the whole body. It increases elasticity of the joints, particularly in the spine. We recommend salute to the sun as a daily warm-up to lead off your yoga routine. While doing salute to the sun, attention should be focused on the breathing and on whatever part of the body seems to be particularly affected at the time. This exercise provides a good overall stretch and also promotes agility and alertness.

Instructions: Okay, now stand up with your feet about shoulder width apart. Take a deep, slow breath into the abdomen. Let it all out and check yourself out. Are you relaxed in the neck, shoulders, back, arms, torse, buttocks, legs, upper and lower and down to your feet? Bring your hands, arms loosely extended, around in front of you, palms in. Lock your thumbs together and extend your fingers.

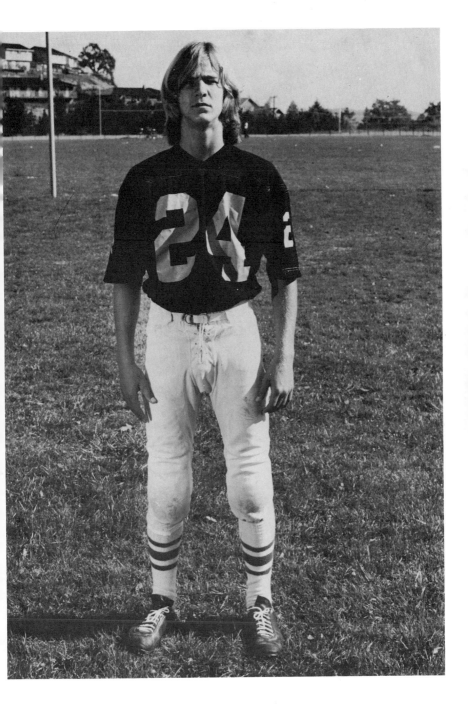

Now bring your hands up, arms extended and directly over your head. Breathe in as you reach up and back. Stretch back as far as you can. Roll your eyes back and try to look at the floor or ground behind you. Stretch until you feel a strain but not a pain. As you practice you'll find you can stretch farther back each week. How much depends on your own body. There is no right amount because as far as you can go, somebody else can go farther. Just do what's right for you and relax and enjoy yourself. Breathe out and bring your arms back over your head and out in front of you. *Did you remember to breathe through your nose?*

Now, keep your knees locked and reach on over to the ground. Put your chin on your chest and stretch out the back of your legs. If your fingers reach the ground, put your palms down. If you can rest on your palms, try to touch with your elbows. Stretch to your own limit.

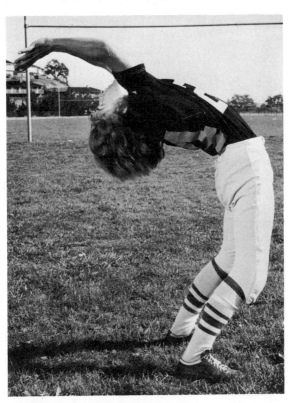

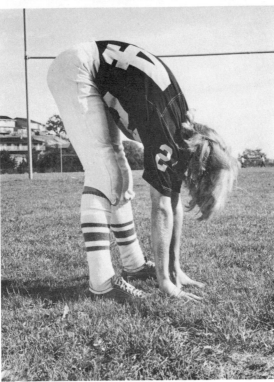

Breathe in and stretch your left leg back as far as possible. Leave your right foot flat on the ground. Reach out with your arms extended to either side of your right knee. Put your chest right down on that right knee. Push the extended left knee down toward the ground. Hold it, with head arched so that the back of your head is touching your back, then exhale.

Now, extend your right leg back with your left. Push your butt up in the air and form a triangle with straight arms and legs bent at the waist. Breathe in and try to slowly push your heels back to the ground. Breathe out now as you let your body come straight and your arms lower your body to the ground. Place your toes together, heels out as you lie on your belly with your hands

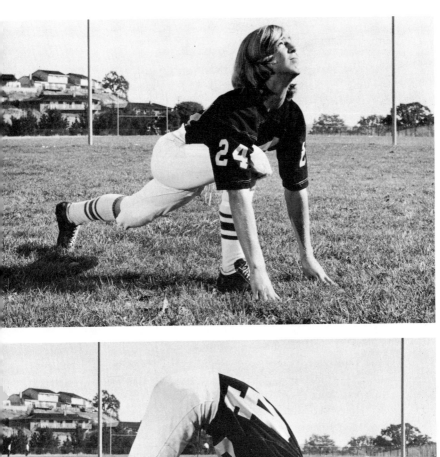

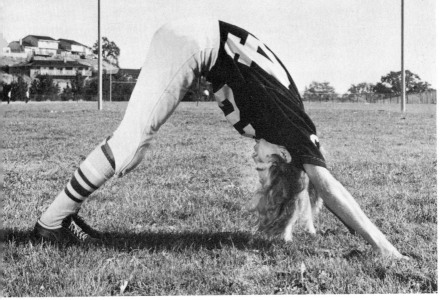

under your shoulders. Now breathe in and push your upper body up off the floor until your arms are fully extended.

First the head goes up, then the chest, then the stomach. Try to keep your pelvis on the ground. Bend your head and neck back as far as possible and roll your eyes up and back in your head. Hold it and concentrate on pushing your hips down to the ground. You should feel this one at the tip of your spine if you've done it right. If not, you'll get it with practice.

Now, let your breath out and let your arms roll your body slowly down to the ground again.

Breathe in again and form another triangle like you did earlier by pushing your butt up in the air. Put your chin on your chest and push your heels down so your feet are as flat on the ground as you can get them.

Breathe out as you bring your left knee forward up under your chest, foot flat on the ground. Leave your right leg extended. Look up and back, press down with the right knee and breathe in.

Breathe out as you come to a squatting position and breathe in and stretch your head and shoulders back. Straighten your legs and arms, leaving your hands on the ground as you did earlier. Breathe out and put your chin on your chest.

Hook your thumbs together and breathe in as you straighten up and stretch up and back over your head with arms extended. Reach and look back as far as you can. Breathe out and bring your hands, arms extended, back to the front of your body and down to your sides. This exercise can be repeated several times if desired, and with practice.

There are two things to concentrate on while doing a yoga exercise. The first is the sound and feel of your breathing. The other is to concentrate on the specific muscles that are tightened or stretched by the exercise. Try to keep your mind clear of all other thoughts. This is an excellent drill for concentration. We tell the players that if their minds start to drift away onto something else, they should remind their minds gently to come back and concentrate on the exercises.

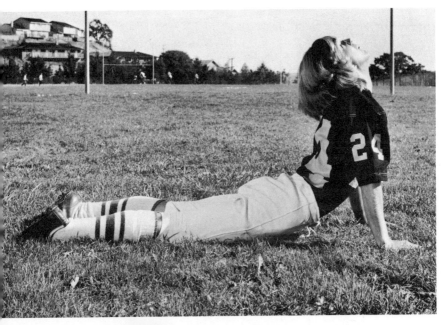

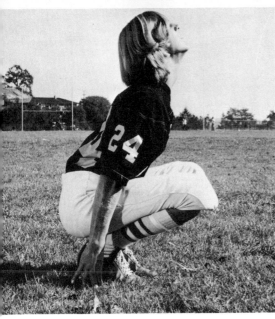

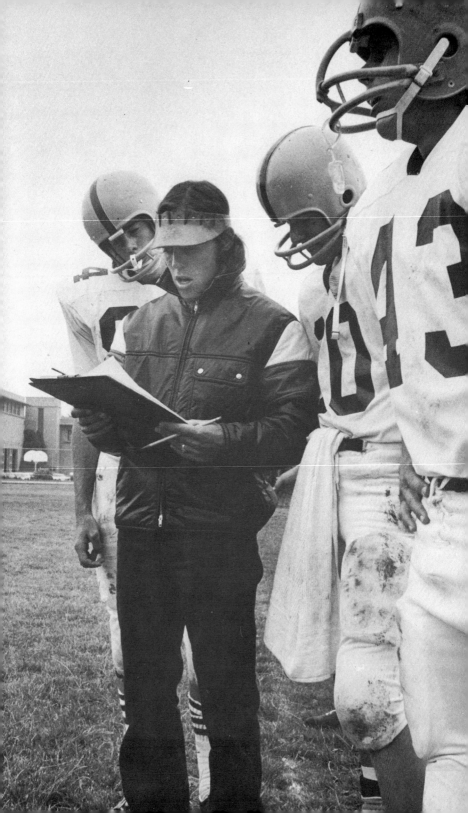

4

The Inverted Postures

The exercises in this chapter are called inverted postures by some
yoga teachers.

Exercise: Shoulder Stand

Benefits: I find that inverted postures, particularly shoulder stands, are good for preventing and healing muscle pulls in the legs, especially groin injuries. If you were at one of our practices, you would often see players with slight leg problems doing shoulder stands on the sides of the field.

This asana is energizing to legs, especially when players have spent much of the day standing round, walking and sitting in class. Like the salute to the sun, the shoulder stand helps to get us going, to get us ready to expend the energy necessary for playing football. It serves to tone us up from the more sedentary activities of the day. Thus, we do shoulder stands early in the exercise period.

While you are in a shoulder stand you should concentrate on breathing, on any sore or strained muscles or tendons in the legs, and on the feel of the blood flowing down the legs which seems to carry away tension, soreness and tiredness.

Instructions: You start a shoulder stand lying on your back. Breathe in a full, deep abdominal breath and breathe it all back out again. Relax as you exhale, through the nose, of course. Now on the next incoming breath, raise the legs and trunk slowly from the ground. Place your hands high on your back and sort of walk them up towards the shoulder blades, bringing the torso and legs higher and straighter. Press your chest onto your chin. Try to rest the weight of your body on the tops of your shoulders and back of your head. Support your body with the hands on your back, elbows on the ground, push waist forward. Now hold it and practice abdominal breathing, slowly and deeply through the nose. Feel the blood coming down your legs. We hold this exercise for at least one minute and as much as three minutes later in the season. Now come back down slowly, rolling each vertebra down one at a time. Just lay on your back, palms up, and breathe. After a few deep breaths, perhaps one or two, you're ready to go to a variation called the Plow.

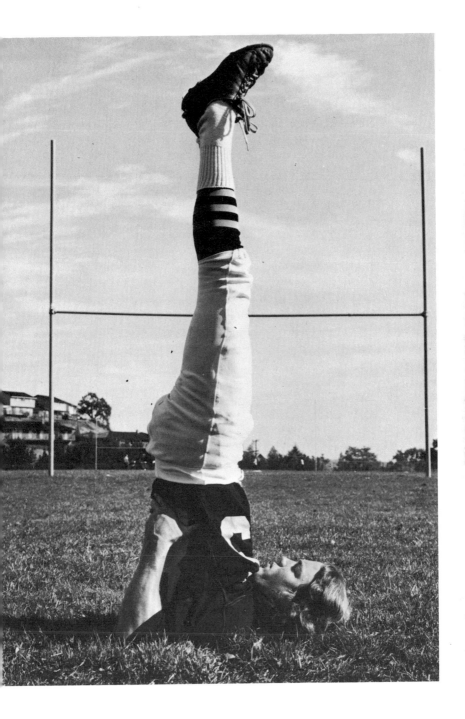

Exercise: Plow

Benefits: This posture, which can be done after holding a shoulder stand for a while, adds to the benefits of the shoulder stand and strengthening of the abdominal muscles. The plow also stretches the vertebra apart and lengthens and smooths the great muscles in the back. The plow loosens and strengthens the cervical area of the spine which is an area in which serious football injuries sometimes occur.

In addition to attending to keeping the breath smooth and deep as possible, you should focus on feeling the back and leg muscles stretch and relax while doing this exercise.

Instructions: Start as in a shoulder stand, on your back, hands at your sides. Bring your legs up, support your back with your hands and try to touch the ground as far beyond your head as possible with your toes. If you touch easily, then walk the toes out above the head until the maximum stretch is achieved. Again, hold it and breathe slowly through the nose and very deeply. Concentrate on the back and leg muscles. If at first you can't reach the ground, keep the legs straight, reach out as far as you can. In time your back and legs will stretch enough to let you reach the ground.

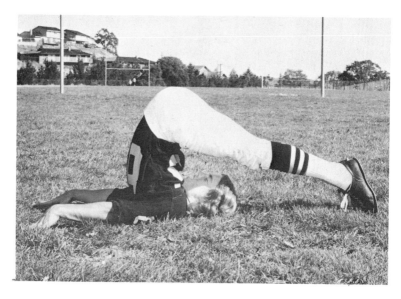

30

Exercise: **Variation of the Plow**

Benefits: Increases the flexibility of the spine, stretches the back muscles and hamstring muscles, strengthens abdominal muscles.

Instructions: Lie on back, arms along the sides with palms down. Raise your legs slowly, bring them over your head lifting from the hip. Gradually lower the toes to the floor, keeping your legs together. Bend the knees and bring them close to your ears.

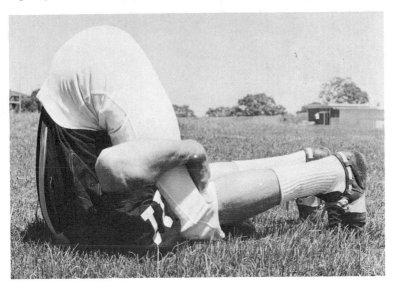

31

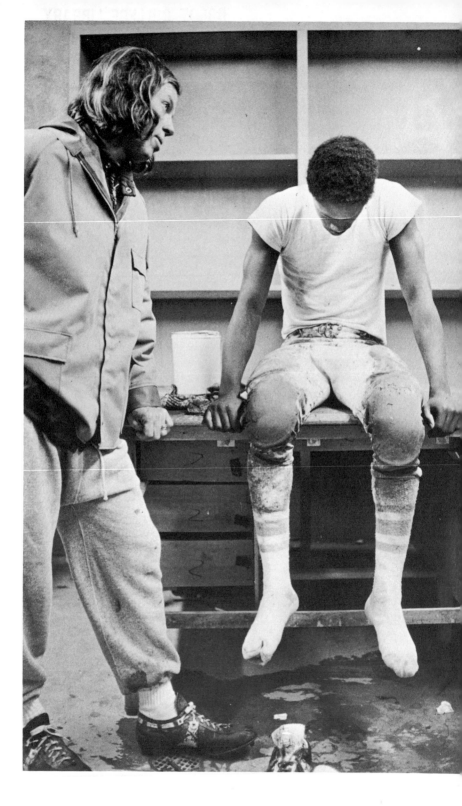

5

Stretching Exercises

As we mentioned earlier, one of the things yoga does for your body is make the muscles long and smooth. In this chapter we will discuss some stretching exercises which we use on a regular basis to protect the bodies of our players from injury. For the most part, these exercises are directed at specific parts of the body, we have organized them so they move from top to bottom.

Exercise: Neck Stretcher

Benefits: This exercise may have saved the life of one of our players. He got involved in a contact with his head down and suffered a neck injury. The player reported to us that without yoga conditioning the injury might have been much worse.

The exercise benefits the neck and shoulder area. Except for the breathing and emphasis on relaxation, it isn't that different from an exercise commonly used by coaches.

Try to relax completely during this exercise and listen for your vertebra to crack.

Instructions: Stand with your feet slightly apart, chin on your chest, arms loosely at your sides. On an incoming abdominal breath move your head slowly, keeping the chin on your chest so that it rotates around and rests on the right shoulder. Rest your cheek on your right shoulder. Rotate to your right again so that your head is all the way back. The back of your head should touch your back. Slowly rotate on until your left cheek rests on your left shoulder and finally you rotate to the starting position. Now repeat the process going the other way, or rotating your head to the left. Relax the neck completely during this exercise. Repeat the exercise going both ways at least three times.

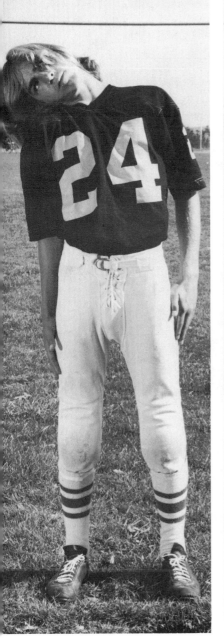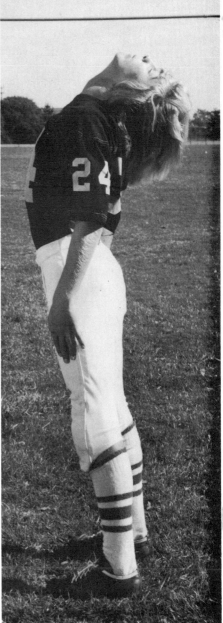

Exercise: **Side Stretcher**

Benefits: This exercise strengthens and relaxes muscles on the sides of the torso and also strengthens the shoulder muscles. This is where the attention should be focused.

Instructions: Start by standing relaxed with your hands loosely hanging at the sides. Bring your hands around to the front of your body and lace the fingers together. Now, keeping your arms extended, stretch up with an incoming breath. Reach as high as you can with your palms up and back behind the head and exhale. Now inhale and stretch to the left, bending at the waist, keeping your legs straight. Exhale as you come to the center and stretch to the right on the next incoming breath. Repeat slowly with the maximum comfortable stretch about three times to both sides. Remember, breathe through the nose. Relax and do at least one inhale and exhale with each exercise.

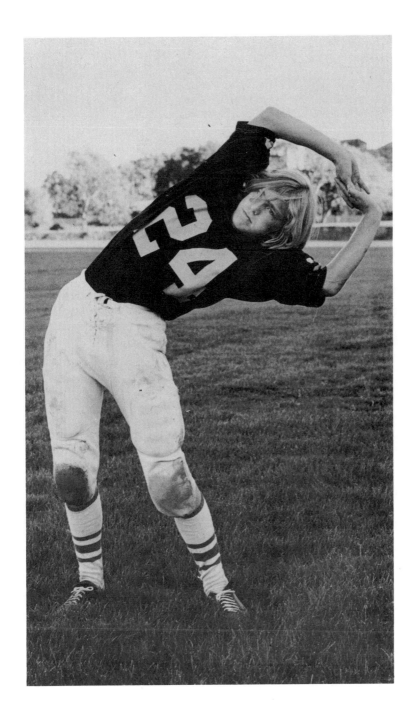

Exercise: Flight

Benefits: This exercise is particularly good for stretching the shoulders, neck, small of the back and thighs. The whole body gets involved.

Instructions: Start by breathing in deeply as you raise your arms in a V over your head, stretch the arms pull them back, and bend over backwards at about 45°. Roll your eyes back and look for the ground over your head. Push your stomach out.

Now exhale as you come back the other way. Bend forward from the waist. Push your chest out as you go down. Press your chin onto your chest. Leave your arms out and press them backward over your head as you go forward. Breathe in as you come up and repeat about four times.

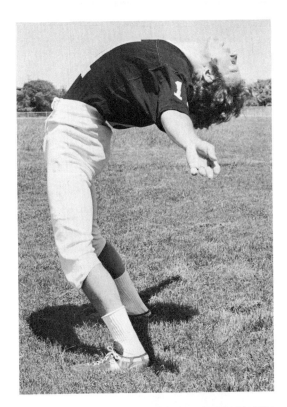

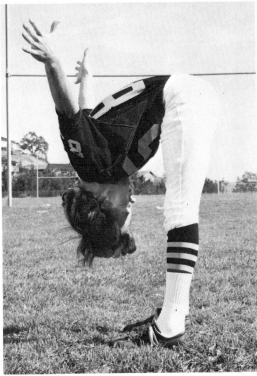

Exercise: **Head Knee Bend**

Benefits: This exercise keeps flexibility of the spine, circulation in the back and stretches the hamstring muscles.

Instructions: Stand upright, bend down slowly pushing your chest out as you bend; then hold your ankles, chin on your chest, keep the legs straight and bring your chest and head as close to your legs as possible. Breathe in as you start to bend forward, hold the position a few seconds, exhale and return to upright position.

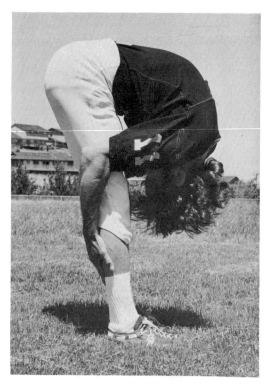

Exercise: **Ankle Grasp**

Benefits: This exercise is directed toward the muscles and tendons at the back of the legs. Hamstring injuries are frequently a problem in football. With this exercise and the others we recommend for the legs, they can be all but eliminated. On our team we just don't get many leg injuries in the first place and those we do get respond quickly to yoga conditioning.

Instructions: Stand with legs a shoulder width apart. Bring your hands around in front and lock the thumbs together. Now on an incoming breath and with your chin on your chest reach around the outside of the left leg and down to the left ankle with both hands. Grasp your ankle and exhale. Come up on the next incoming breath and repeat the same move to the right side. Stretch to both sides about three times. It is important to keep your legs straight and your knees locked in this exercise.

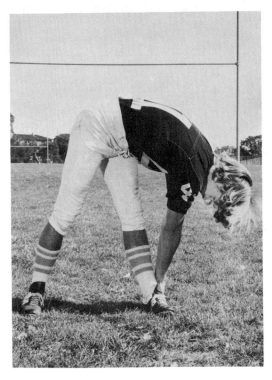

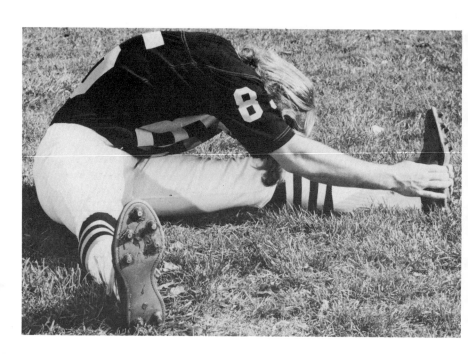

Exercise: **Leg Split**

Benefits: Many of the exercises we recommend on first glance don't appear to be that different from calisthenics that have been used for decades by football and track coaches. The main difference is in emphasis and mental attitude about the exercise. When we get into a posture in yoga we relax, breathe deeply and concentrate on the part of the body that is being affected. The emphasis is never on straining; rather, we concentrate on relaxing and stretching.

In this exercise, the hamstring muscles and particularly the sides and back of the knees are affected.

Instructions: Starting in a sitting position with your legs stretched out at a 45° angle from each other, lock your thumbs together and stretch your arms high over your head with an incoming breath. Keep both legs flat on the ground and reach out for the left foot. Bend at the waist, not in the back. Push the chest out as you are going down. Try to bring the chest out to your knee. Grasp your foot by wrapping your fingers around it. Put your forehead down on your knee and exhale. Relax and concentrate on your stretched out leg muscles.

Check out your legs. Are your knees locked and legs flat on the ground? If not, grasp the ankles as far down as you can reach, or bend the foot back towards you and grasp the toes. Now relax and breathe into your abdomen. You may find you can stretch another inch or so on each exhalation. About three breath cycles is enough. On an incoming breath come up to the hand over head position and reach out along the right leg.

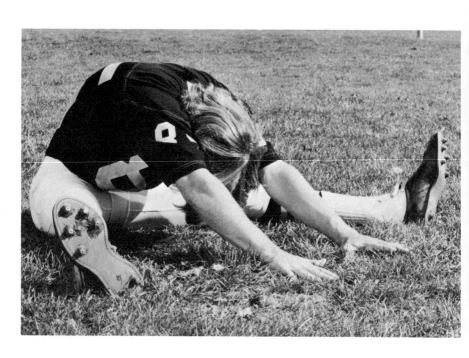

Exercise: Between the Legs Stretch

Benefits: The emphasis shifts to the upper leg, buttocks and small of the back in this exercise.

Instructions: Now reach out between the legs from the same sitting posture with hands over the head. Place the hands flat on the ground. Push the chest out and down. Concentrate on the breath and relax.

Groin injuries have been a major problem in all types of athletics. The next few pages include five different exercises you can do to stretch and strengthen the groin area and the muscles of the inner leg. It is important to start slowly; use your own judgment on how far you can stretch this area. By mixing these exercises daily and holding each position five seconds, I feel you can come very close to eliminating all groin injuries. In the three years I have been using these groin exercises we have not had a person miss a game because of a groin injury. When starting to use these exercises, you may feel sore and stiff in the groin area, but as I mentioned earlier the shoulder stand or head stand is an excellent exercise to heal that area.

Exercise: Standing Groin Stretcher

Benefits: To strengthen and stretch muscles of the groin area and the muscles of the inner leg.

Instructions: Start with your feet about shoulder width apart. Inhale as you stretch over to the left ankle with the left hand. Let the right hand curve up over the head, keeping both legs straight. Exhale and stand up. Then work to the other side. Concentrate on the groin area.

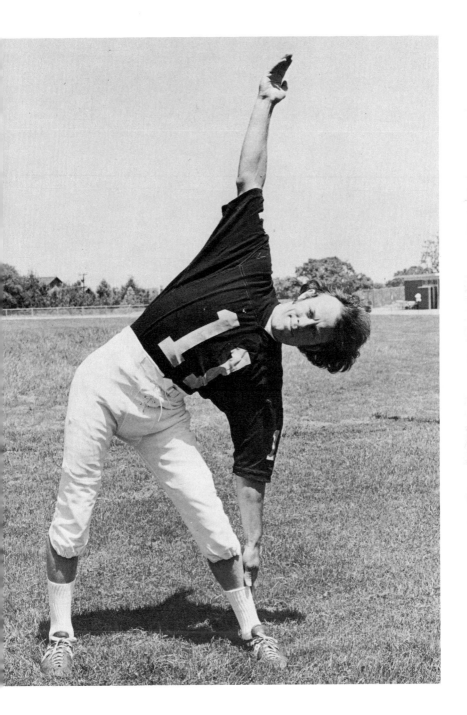

Exercise: **Kneeling Groin Stretcher**

Benefits: To strengthen and stretch muscles of the groin area and the muscles of the inner leg.

Instructions: Start with your right knee on the ground extending the left leg straight out to the side. Inhale as you stretch to the left ankle with the left hand. Keep the back straight, let the right hand curve up over the head. Exhale and relax, then work to the other side. Concentrate on the groin area.

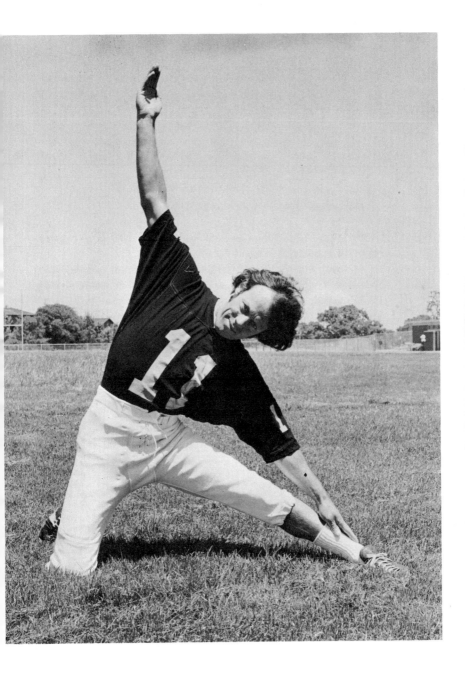

Exercise: Bend Knee Groin Stretcher

Benefits: To strengthen and stretch muscles of the groin area and the muscles of the inner leg.

Instructions: Bend your right leg at knee and extend your left leg out to the side. Inhale as you stretch over to the left ankle with the left hand. Keep your back straight, let your right hand curve up over the head. Exhale and relax, then work to the other side. Concentrate on the groin area.

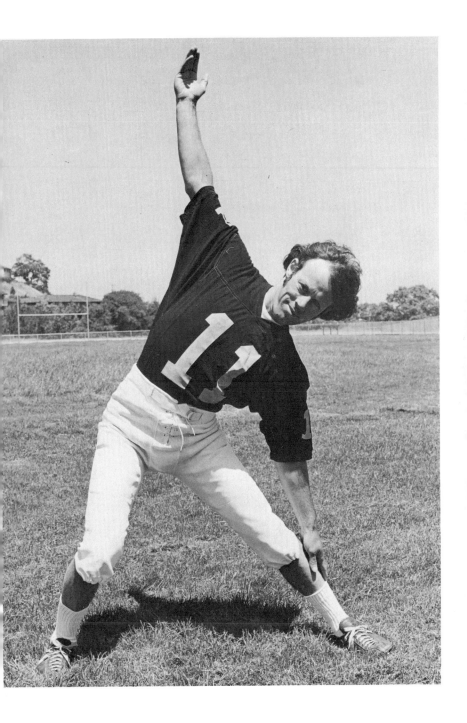

Exercise: **Squat Groin Stretcher**

Benefits: To strengthen and stretch muscles of the groin area and the muscles of the inner leg.

Instructions: Start with both feet pointed out to the sides, keep your back straight, arms out to the side, and squat down. Hold your knees out to the side as you squat down. Inhale as you squat down; exhale as you come up. A variation of this exercise is to squat down and instead of coming all the way up, come about six inches, hold, then down again.

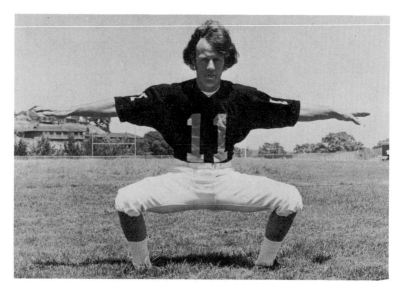

Exercise: **Splits Groin Stretcher**

Benefits: To strengthen and stretch muscles of the groin area and the muscles of the inner leg.

Instructions: Spread both legs out to the side, feet are out to the side also. Keep your legs straight, try and do the splits using your hands for balance.

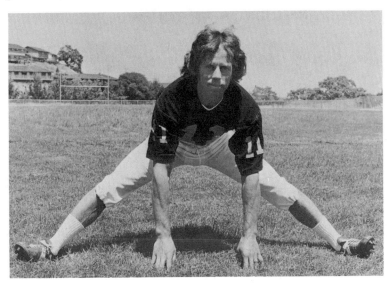

Exercise: Foot Inside Thigh Stretch

Benefits: Again, this is a leg exercise. It stretches the lower part of the thigh, stretches the knee area and the lower back.

Instructions: This stretcher starts by putting one foot, say the left, high up on your right thigh while sitting on the ground with your leg extended flat. This is called the foot inside thigh stretch. Again start with your hands coming up over your head as you inhale deeply through the nose. Now reach out as far as you can pushing the chest out and down and grasp the right foot or ankle. Exhale and relax. Then inhale, come back up and try it on the other side.

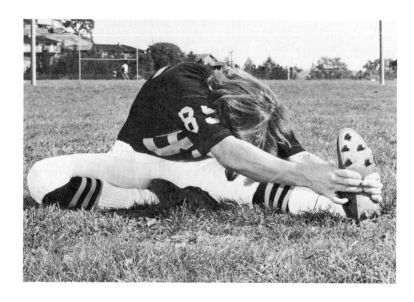

Exercise: **Legs Together Stretch**

Benefits: This exercise is also a variation on the forward stretching exercises. Again, emphasis is on the leg muscles and lower back.

Instructions: This variation involves putting your legs together flat on the ground, reach out and place your hands under your calves and push your chest out and down, placing your head on your knees and elbows on the ground.

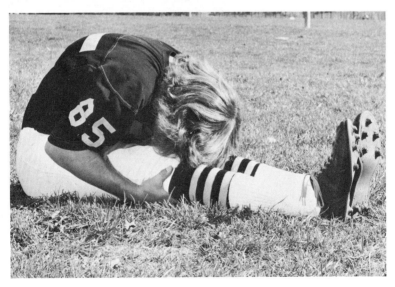

55

Exercise: **Ankle Exercise**

Benefits: Improves circulation in the lower leg and foot, which serves to prevent injury and promote healing.

Instructions: Start in a sitting position, raise one leg so that your foot is about 6 inches from the ground. Curl your toes under and bend your foot away from you towards the ground. Breathe in and hold for five seconds and relax. Repeat with the other foot.

Next raise your foot again and stretch your toes back towards your knee. Hold for five seconds again and relax. Repeat with the other foot.

Stretch your foot to the right next using the same hold and relax routine. Then stretch to the left.

A variation on this exercise involves raising your foot six inches from the ground and rotating in a circle first one way and then the other. Concentrate on breathing in while rotating and on the feel of your ankle.

Exercise: **Ankle Lifts**

Benefits: Promotes circulation in the ankles and strengthens them.

Instructions: Start in a standing position. Keeping your toes together, turn your heels out as far as possible. Breathe in and come up on your toes. Breathe out, relax and come down. Repeat ten to fifteen times. Next, place your heels together and toes out. Breathe in and come up on your toes, relax, breathe out and slowly come down again. Again, repeat ten to fifteen times.

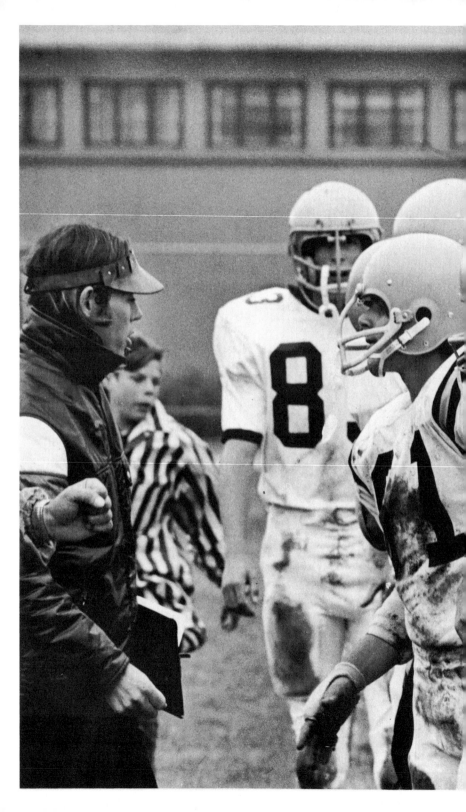

6

Torso Exercises

Contact sports require concentration. Football requires knowledge and skill, but strength is also important. In the human body the origin of strength for large muscle activities like blocking, tackling and running is in the torso. The large muscles of the abdomen and chest and the long muscles of the back are the base for the movement. The stronger these large muscles are the more powerful that player's moves will be.

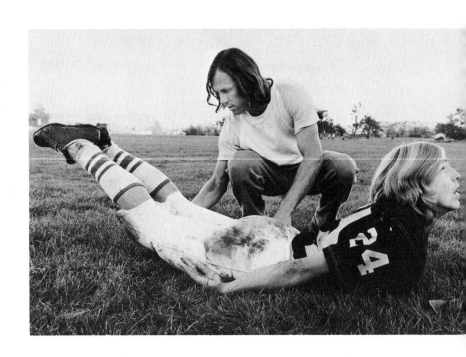

Exercise: **The Swing**

Benefits: This exercise, which is a variation on the locust, tightens and works the shoulders in addition to the hips and back.

Instructions: Get down on your belly, arms by your side. On an incoming breath, raise your feet and legs and your arms at the same time. Hold it for a slow five count and slowly and gently come down as you exhale.

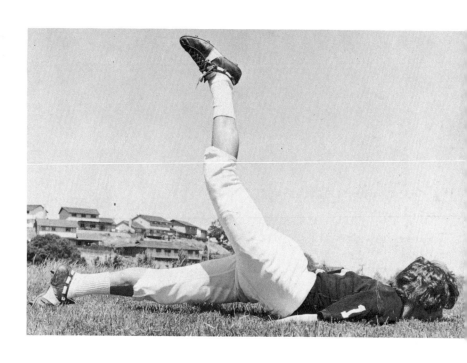

Exercise: Half Locust

Benefits: Strengthens the muscles of the lower back, shoulders, abdomen and hamstring muscles.

Instructions. Lie prone on ground, keep your hands alongside your body, make fists and put them under your thighs or along the sides. Take a deep breath, stiffen your leg, keeping your toe pointed and lift one leg as high as you can; hold it five to ten seconds while holding the breath. Exhale and let your leg down slowly. Do the same with your other leg.

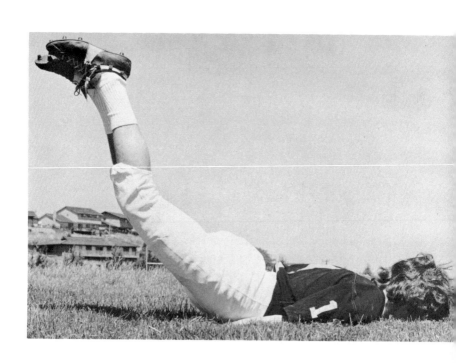

Exercise: Full Locust

Benefits: Strengthens the muscles of the lower back, shoulders, abdomen and hamstring muscles.

Instructions: Lie prone on the ground and keep your hands alongside your body. Take a deep breath, stiffen your body, supporting yourself on the chest and hands. Lift your legs as high as you can, hold it five to ten seconds while holding your breath. Exhale and let your legs down slowly.

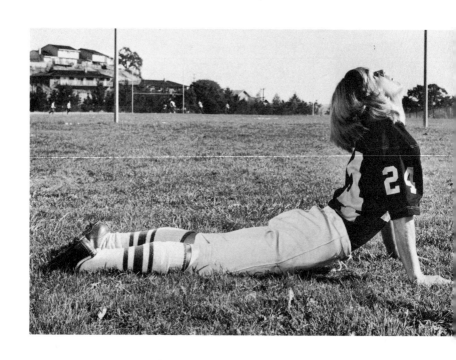

Exercise: Cobra

Benefits: This exercise makes the spine more flexible and strengthens the back and abdominal muscles as well.

Instructions: Start with your hands, palms down, near or under the shoulders. Now point your toes in and let your heels roll out. Push your body up slowly and arch the back and neck. Come up with your head first then your chest and stomach. When your arms are fully extended, push out your stomach. Try to touch your back with the back of your head. Feel the pressure on your spine as you are going up to the cobra. Come down slowly, keep your head on your back as you come down.

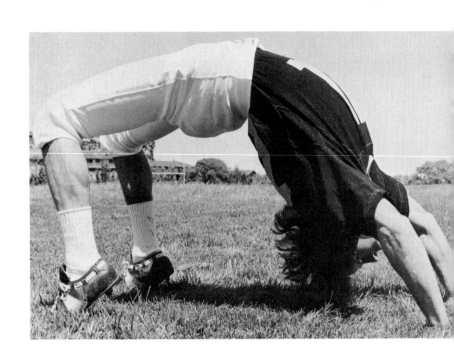

Exercise: **The Wheel**

Benefits: This exercise provides a tremendous stretch of the spine and its associated ligaments. The effect is fairly general. Shoulders, chest, abdomen and lower back are also involved.

Instruction: Start on your back with the knees bent, legs slightly apart and feet flat on the ground. Place your arms over your head with your hands palms down fingers pointing back toward the shoulders. Now raise your heels off the ground and lift your body up as high as possible. When you get up, bring your head back toward your feet. Hold it for 15 seconds and come down slowly and gently.

Exercise: **Variation of the Wheel**

Benefits: Bending and stretching of the legs, hips, shoulders, chest and arms.

Instructions: Bring your feet up to the buttock, feet apart, and place your hands on either side of your head, palms down with fingers toward your shoulders. Breathe in and push up into a bridge, lifting your body as high as possible off the floor. Lift your left leg, pointing your toe as high as possible. Another variation, lift your left arm along with the left leg. This variation is excellent for balance and flexibility.

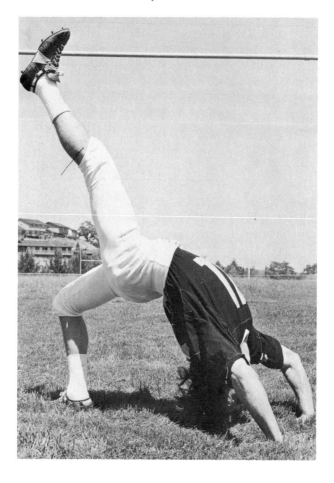

Exercise: **The Half Bow**

Benefits: The half bow and the full bow are particularly useful for stretching the abdominal area, hip area and the thighs and upper back.

Instructions: From the prone down position extend your left hand back and grasp the left ankle by bending at the left knee. Extend the right arm and leg. Now hang onto your left ankle and raise your right hand as your body bends up in a bow on an incoming breath. Exhale as you come back down. Press out with your leg and bring your head back for the full benefit. Try it on the other side too.

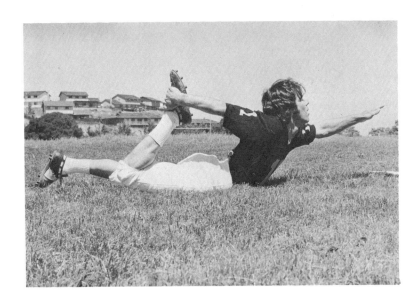

Exercise: **The Full Bow**

Benefits: The areas affected are the same as in the half bow, but this asana is considerably more difficult than the one-sided version described above.

Instruction: Start on your belly again. Bring up both ankles. Reach back and grab first one and then the other. Arch up, bring your head back and press hard against your hands with your legs. Breathe in as you go up, out as you come gently down. Hold it for about ten seconds.

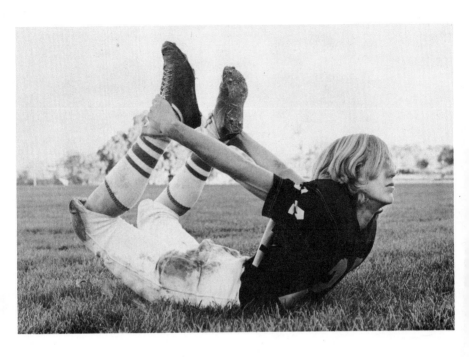

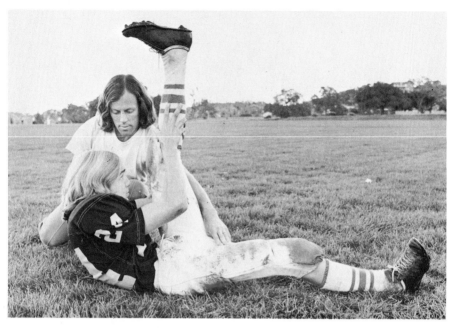

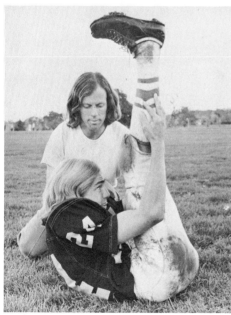

Exercise: Chest to Knee Stretch

Benefits: This exercise works on the torso as the other asanas in this chapter do, but it also provides a stretch for the Achilles tendons, hamstrings, calf muscles, upper back and neck.

Instructions: Start by laying on your back. With an incoming breath raise your right leg slowly. Keep your leg straight. Bend the toes back toward your head and you will feel it pulling along the back of your leg. Grasp the back of your leg with your hands and raise your body and stretch the chest and head towards your knee. The body comes to the leg rather than the leg to the body.

Try it with the left leg then with both legs together.

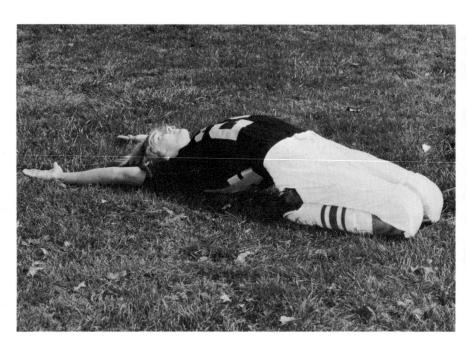

Exercise: Camel

Benefits: Most people really feel this exercise in the upper thighs and ankles as well as the abdomen. It is also said to stimulate the thyroid gland and promote the filtering of impurities out of the body.

Instructions: The camel starts by you sitting on your heels with your legs tucked under you, knees together. Now breathe in as you bend backwards, first onto your right elbow then on your left. Finally, back onto your head. If that's too easy, go all the way to your back, but keep the knees together and on the ground. Now relax and concentrate on your breathing. You can stretch your arms out past your head or place them on your thighs. Come up slowly, using your right or left elbow to help you up.

Exercise: **Variation of the Camel**

Benefits: Thigh muscles and shoulder muscles stretched, stomach muscles fully stretched.

Instructions: Sit on your knees, bend back keeping your thighs straight, push your stomach out putting both hands flat on the floor. Lower your head as much as you can. Breathe in as you go back, hold a few seconds, exhale and relax.

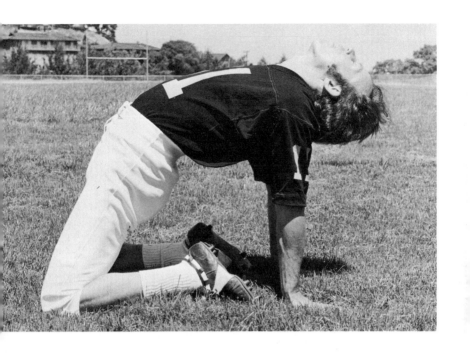

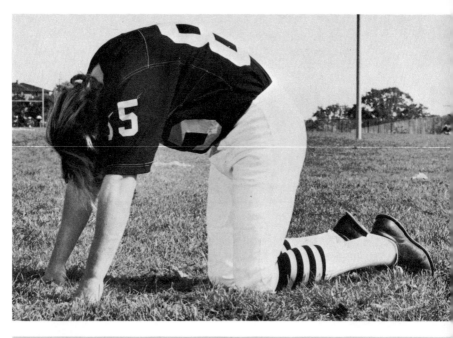

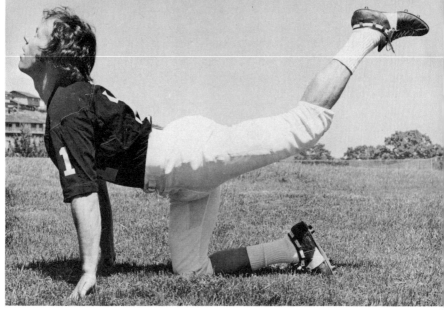

Exercise: The Cat

Benefits: This exercise is somewhat less demanding of physical strength than the other asanas in this chapter. Yet still it provides a good stretch of the upper and lower back and hamstrings.

Instruction: Start on your hands and knees with the legs slightly apart. On an incoming breath, stretch the head back as far as you can, let your stomach sag towards the floor.

Then, extend the leg out behind you as far as you can reach with the toe pointed. Hold it for about ten seconds. Return slowly to the hands and knees position. Then put your chin on your chest, arch your back up as high as you can and hold that. Repeat the process using the other leg.

Exercise: Feet to Hand

Benefits: This exercise works the shoulders, middle and lower back and, when the toes are curled back properly, the whole back of the legs as well.

Instructions: Start on your back with your arms spread to the sides, palms up. On an incoming breath raise both legs, keeping them together and straight. Try to keep the toes curled up toward the head. Keeping the right shoulder on the ground, move your legs over to the extended left hand. When you've reached as far as you can, breathe out, relax and on the next incoming breath return your legs to the original position and repeat to the other side. Move slowly and gently, being careful to lower your back to the ground carefully.

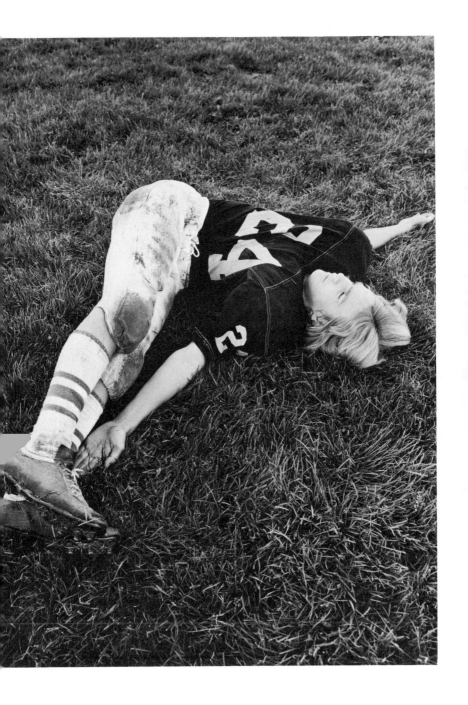

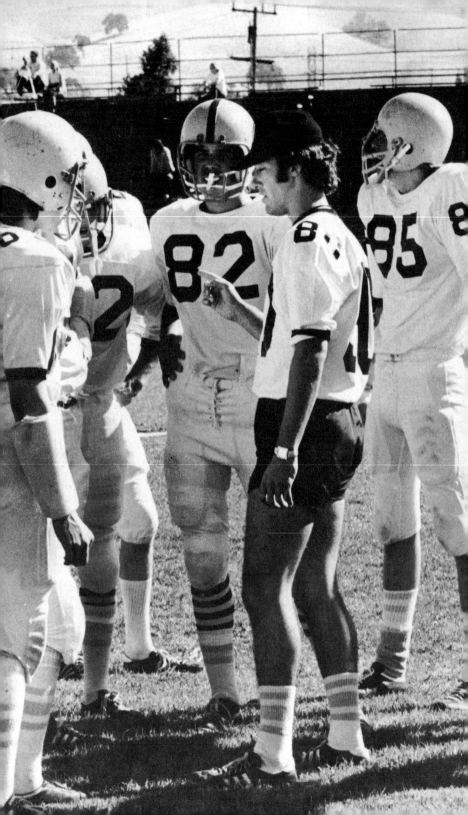

7

Balance Exercises

Balance is an important part of any contact sport. In football it is important for offensive backs and receivers as well as for defensive secondary players. It is equally important with a different emphasis for linemen. Yoga offers some exercises that seem particularly well suited to gaining a good sense of balance.

Exercise: **Flying Stork**

Benefits: Balance, flexibility, exercises the leg muscles.
Instructions: Grab your right ankle, pulling your leg as close to the buttocks as possible. Put your left arm straight up. Concentrate on abdominal breathing. Do the same with the other leg and arm.

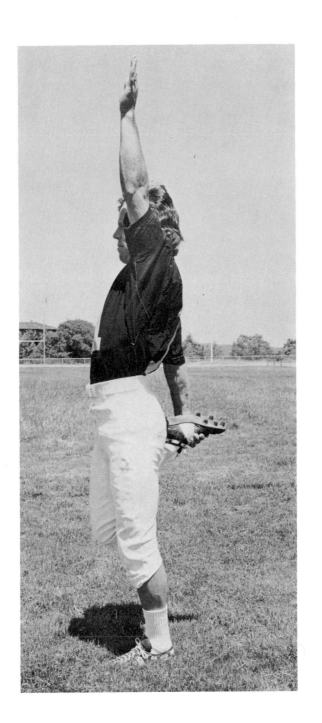

Exercise: **Variation Flying Stork**

Benefits: Balance, flexibility, exercises the leg muscles and stretches various ligaments.

Instructions: Pull your knee and ankle up as high as you can pushing out with the foot. Lean forward slightly and raise arm up high as possible and head back.

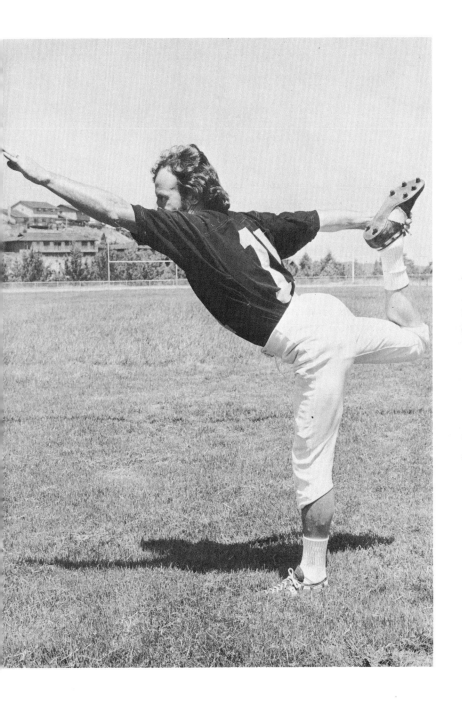

Exercise: **One Foot Squat**

Benefits: This is probably the balance exercise that requires the most composure and concentration of those we have presented. It is particularly good for linemen since they work out of a more compact stance like the squatting position.

Instructions: Squat on your toes. Put one hand down for balance and use the other to pull your left foot up and rest it on your right thigh. Now carefully bring the palms of your hands together, fingers up in front of your chest. Oops! Well, try it again. It helps to look off at the horizon on this one and, of course, concentrate on your breathing and relax. Again, work on both sides. If one side seems harder than the other, then work more on that side.

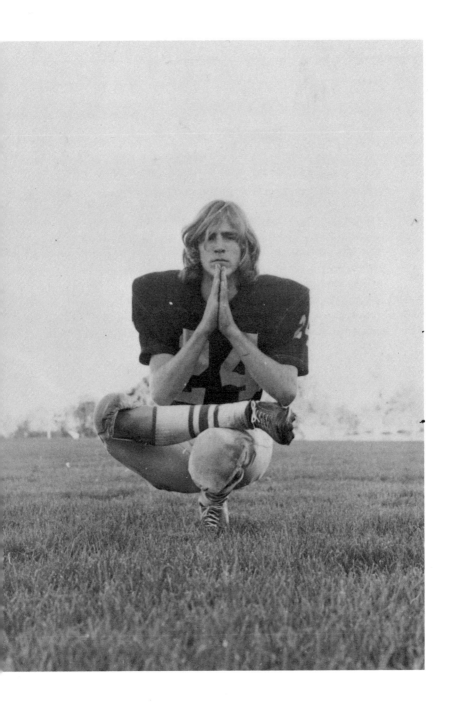

Exercise: **Sponge or Corpse Pose**

Benefits: This pose is for relaxation at the end of the session. It lets the value of the exercise set in, it also has a calming effect on the nerves; and will help to relax unnecessary tension on the muscles.

Instructions: Lie on your back, hands by your side with palms up and feet apart, heels pointed in and toes out. You can use any of the three breathing exercises I have mentioned: abdominal, complete breath or alternate breathing in this position. Concentrate only on the breath, remember if the mind starts to wander away to something else bring it back gently to the breathing exercise. I usually start with abdominal breathing an then use one of the other two to finish the exercise. 3 to 10 minutes.

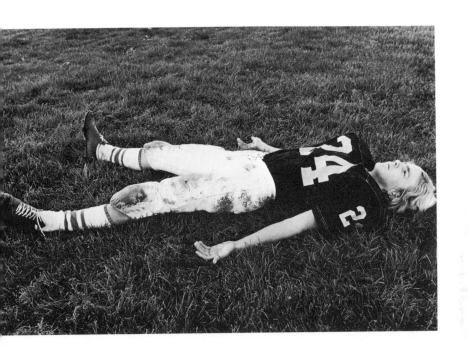

Yoga and football—what a combination! Yoga is a science that teaches you to relax and slow you down as well as bring you closer to knowing yourself. Yoga gives you a feeling of calmness and peace of mind. Football is a game of tackling, blocking, running and knocking an opponent down. I have attempted to show how an Eastern discipline, Hatha Yoga, can benefit people who are interested in football and other sports.

For twenty-two years I have been involved in football as a player and as a coach. Football is a beautiful game, it is a game of skill, coordination, balance, concentration, conditioning, grace and togetherness. As players and as coaches we all learn how to lose and how to win. We have to learn to accept both of these experiences. As in life, we are successful in many of the things we do, but there are times when we fail. I feel through sports one can learn to accept failure by learning from the mistakes made. With that understanding we all try not to let the same mistake be made over again, so we profit by this failure, realizing this is a lesson learned. While participating in sports at any level, the experience that we receive is a tremendous lesson in life.

As a teacher it is important to develop a togetherness among team members. The togetherness we talk about is brotherhood. We practice together, we play together, we share together, we win together, we lose together and most important we LOVE one another.

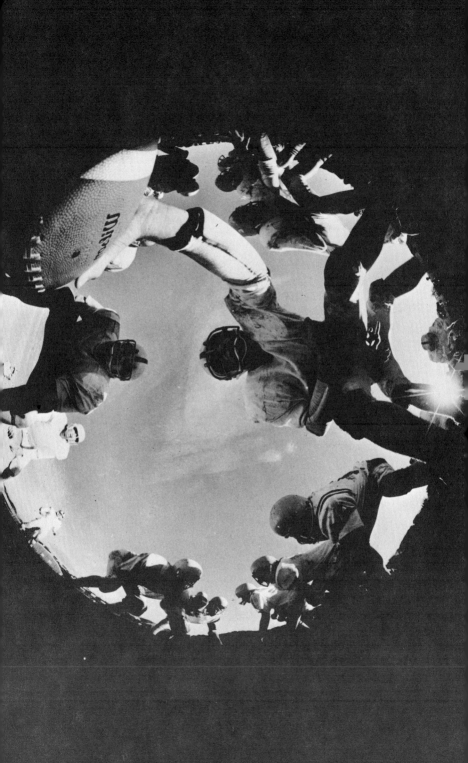

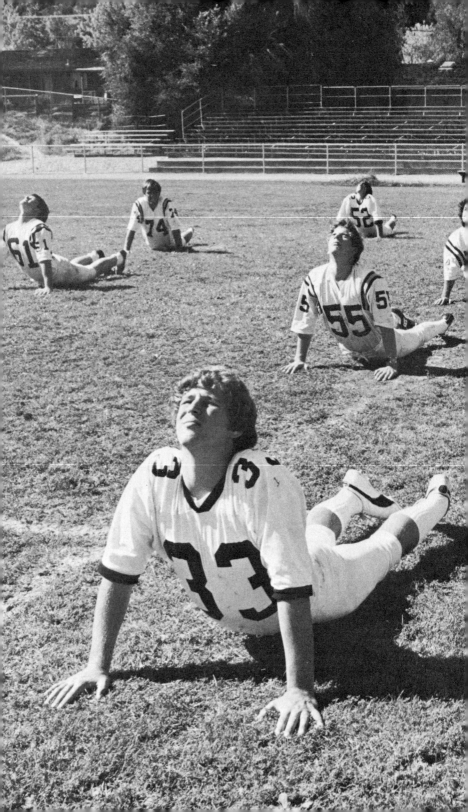

8

Yoga Conditioning and Sport

In this book some hatha yoga exercises and techniques are discussed as a conditioning method for football. It is my belief that hatha yoga can play a part in the conditioning of participants in all other sports. The rest of this chapter is devoted to some of the more general benefits of hatha yoga conditioning using episodes from my own athletic experience as examples.

All my life I have believed in the beauty of sports. It started when I was seven years old. The recreation department in my hometown offered tennis lessons for kids and I took them. The next year I played Little League baseball. I continued playing baseball through Babe Ruth League. I also continued to play tennis on the high school tennis team and a year on the tennis team in junior college.

When I was a freshman in high school I weighed 98 lbs., but I went out for football anyway. The coach tried to cut me, but I went to him in tears and convinced him of my determination to play. I got a uniform. When we were dressing for road games and I heard the coach call my name, I knew it was because some other player had forgotten a piece of equipment and the coach wanted to give him mine.

I was manager for varsity basketball during my freshman year in high school so that I could be involved with the sport. In my junior year I played in the preliminary games in football and came back as a cheerleader for the varsity game.

Sports have played a big role in my life. They have been a major part of my education in the sense that what happened to me as a school boy athlete surely has had an influence on me as an adult and as a teacher. For example, my experiences in high school have made the decision to drop a player from my team the hardest decision I have to make as a coach. If I have a uniform for a boy, I will not drop him from the team. Sometimes my reluctance to cut players pays off in ways that surprise me. One of the best linebackers in our league is a boy I had cut once and then I reconsidered when he asked me for a second chance.

What does all this past history have to do with yoga? Mostly it goes to show that I was raised in the same, "grit your teeth and try extra hard" tradition as most other American athletes. When I started studying yoga several years ago a new dimension was added to my sports life.

One of the things I find most beautiful about sports is the experience of reaching down into myself for a hidden reserve that supports an extra effort. Maybe you find you are able to run a little faster, or twist and stretch in a new direction or move your body into position with more agility. Yoga conditioning exercises, like the ones we recommend here makes a greater physical and mental effort possible. In addition, the mind control that hatha yoga practice lends an athlete, allows him or her to fully experience the testing of limits that sports and life provide. Many people who practice yoga achieve a kind of stillness of mind that focuses them in the "here and now" and allows them to experience the maximum use of their bodies and minds at play. Sometimes this means feeling pain, but almost every veteran athlete comes to accept pain as an expected and even desirable part of the game.

One interesting example of this sort of experience occurred this past winter when my family went skiing. It was my first trip of the season. On the first few runs I became so absorbed with the techniques of bending my knees just right, planting the pole just right, leaning forward, and unweighting my skis that I actually forgot to enjoy the sport of skiing. I noticed that I wasn't getting any better with all the attention to details and technique. So I just let the details go and got into a flowing, smooth place with my skiing the way I do with yoga. Soon I found myself skiing much better. I was almost as one with the snow and the skis. My movements became rhythmical and seemed slow and very positive.

Many times we waste too much energy, concerning ourselves with technique, form and style. Recreational sports should be enjoyed because they're fun, and any kind of exercise is good for us. If you get caught up in not enjoying yourself, stop and take a few deep breaths, relax and remind yourself of the real purpose of the sport, which is the enjoyment of having fun.

In sports where you practice during the week and prepare yourself for an event, work on your needs to improve. Work on learning to relax so you can have control over yourself. Do not waste energy thinking about past mistakes or thoughts that will distract your attention. It is possible to be totally involved with the flow of the activity. When you are at oneness with the activity, you will be using your maximum potential as a physical, mental and spiritual being.

Another valuable part of sports is the experience of winning and losing in situations in which considerable energy and effort are invested. There is a similarity between the game of life and a sport. Competitive sports provide us with an area in which to rehearse how we might act as winners and losers outside of the sports field. We can also sample the consequences of certain kinds of actions and attitudes.

Athletic competition brings out some of the finest aspects of human nature. Perhaps the most excellent of these is the capacity to recover from defeat with an even greater determination to win, or to improve one's self. A calm and deliberate state of mind is important, both to winning and to profiting from defeat. I believe much progress can be achieved in this state of mind through the practice and study of yoga. It also seems to me that some of the players whom I coach and the students in my physical education classes have made progress in this direction with the yoga techniques which we do together.

A few years ago I was eliminated from a tennis tournament and got so upset that my body was worn out for two days. I made some mistakes early in the match and as the game went on, I used up my energy and determination by berating and cursing at myself. The harder I tried, the more I swore and mumbled to myself. It wasn't long before I had completely defeated myself.

In contrast to this is my recent experience in learning how to play racketball. I concentrated and did abdominal breathing in between points, enjoyed the game and as in every sport, I played

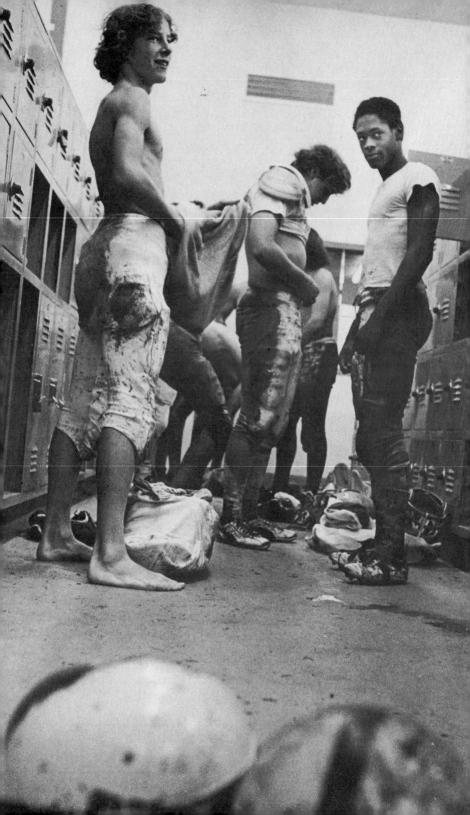

to win. Yet I also was careful to play each point one at a time. Not being concerned with my mistakes. By staying in the "here and now" you can eliminate negative thoughts that distract you from your play.

Remembering myself as a junior college tennis player I shake my head and laugh. One year I broke seven tennis rackets by throwing them on the ground in temper tantrums.

Hatha yoga focus one's attention on the present and calms the spirit and the body in a way that seems to prepare one for a maximum effort. The calm and clear mind can better appreciate the experience of making an effort that pushes the limits of strength, endurance and skill. Good skiers, skilled runners, agile ball players are beautiful to watch. They have a source of flow, grace, and power that often inspires people who attend athletic events.

Yoga is a path that makes available to the sports participant the grace, flow, power and positive attitude. This can be sensed even more completely by the player than by the spectator. These feelings are available to all sports participants from the highly trained and skilled professional athlete to the weekend bicycle enthusiast peddling through the park on Sunday afternoon. We all are beautiful people when we play and yoga is a way to help us get more in touch with our beauty.

In planning a yoga conditioning session it is important to balance the way the body is bent. In the exercises that work to the right or left side of the body we have already suggested that you work to one side and then the other. However, some of the exercises bend the back forward and others bend it back. It is just as important to alternate these exercises so the back isn't always stretched the same way.

Here we will show a chart which outlines a set of exercises which might be selected for use on any given day along with some alternatives. We drew it up bearing in mind the things we have said about the different directions one should bend the body. Many people won't be interested in following a complete yoga program, but I feel if you can utilize some of these exercises to help you in one way or another that is the purpose of this book.

This book is not intended as a complete work on yoga. If you study further you will discover new exercises that seem appropriate to you. We urge you to use them to work out your own program.

DAILY WORKOUT CHART FOR YOGA CONDITIONING

Exercises	Alternatives
* Salute to the sun	Recommended every day
* Shoulder stand	Recommended every day
* Plow	Variation of the plow
* Neck Stretcher	Recommended every day
* Side stretcher	Recommended every day
* Flight	Recommended every day
Head knee bend	Ankle grasp
* Leg split	Between leg stretch
Foot inside thigh stretch	Legs together stretch
* Half locust	Full locust
* Ankle exercise	Ankle lifts
* Cobra	The swing
* Wheel	Variation of the wheel
* Full bow	Half bow
* Chest to knee stretch	Feet to hand
* Camel	Variation of camel
Cat	Recommended every day
Knee bend	One foot squat
* Flying stork	Variation of flying stork
* Standing groin stretcher	Recommended every day
* Kneeling groin stretcher	Bend knee groin stretcher
Squat groin stretcher	Splits groin stretcher
* Sponge or corpse pose	Recommended every day

*Daily exercises that we use with our workout program. As
the season progresses and the players learn these exercises
I will use many of the variations.